SOWING SEEDS

of

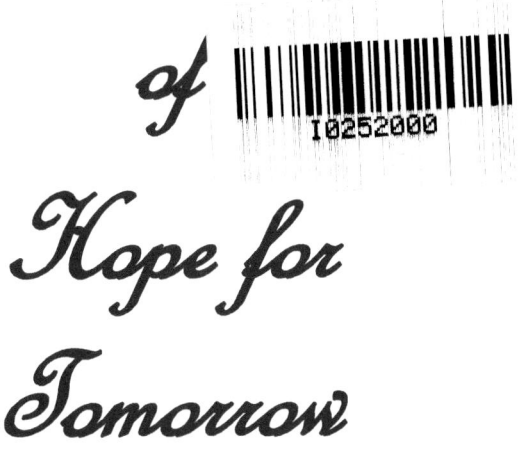

Hope for

Tomorrow

Seven Keys to Restoring Your Sense of Purpose Despite Long-Term Illness

Joanne Bracewell, APRN-C, GS-C

Storehouse Media Group, LLC
Jacksonville, FL

SOWING SEEDS OF HOPE FOR TOMORROW

Copyright © 2019 by Joanne Bracewell

All rights reserved. No part of this book may be used or reproduced by any means, graphic, electronic, or mechanical, including photocopying, recording, taping or by any information storage retrieval system without the written permission of the publisher except in the case of brief quotations embodied in critical articles and reviews.

Books may be ordered through booksellers or by contacting:
Joanne Bracewell
Gracesongmin@gmail.com

The views expressed in this work are solely those of the author and do not necessarily reflect the views of the publisher, and the publisher hereby disclaims any responsibility for them.

Publisher Information:
Storehouse Media Group, LLC
Jacksonville, Florida
Hello@StorehouseMediaGroup.com
www.StorehouseMediaGroup.com

Scripture quotations taken from the New American Standard Bible® (NASB),
Copyright © 1960, 1962, 1963, 1968, 1971, 1972, 1973, 1975, 1977, 1995 by The Lockman Foundation

Used by permission. www.Lockman.org

ISBN: 978-1-943106-43-1 (paperback)
ISBN: 978-1-943106-44-8 (ebook)

Library of Congress Control Number: 2019935868

Printed in the United States of America

Dedication

To my dad.

You were always my inspiration

to succeed at loving others

as Christ has loved me.

"I too have experienced the long-term illness of my mom and how she was a blessing and not a burden. As I read through this book for those who are suffering from sadness and long-term illness, Joanne hit home with the seven keys. She has an encouraging message that no matter what illness or disease one may have, there is still hope, there is still an opportunity for joy and peace to be present in your daily life."

SHERI POWELL
Author of Pausing with God: A Journey Through Menopause, and Pausing in His Presence: a Shut-in Experience
Founder of Pausing with God Ministries,
www.pausingwithgod.com

"As a former nurse and family caregiver, I enjoyed reading Nurse Practitioner Joanne Bracewell's book: *Sowing Seeds of Hope for Tomorrow*. Her concept of hope and renewed purpose in the life of chronically ill people and their caregivers is life-altering. Using seven keys to achieve this change is beautifully presented and God-inspired wisdom."

CAROLYN FAIN SHARP
Former Nurse and caregiver

"This book is a great treasure to anyone willing to serve the hurting in our societies. As a cross-cultural missionary, I find it a great asset in my toolbox."

MISSIONARY PETER WAGURA
Founder and Director, Alive to Serve
www.alivetoserve.org

"This little book addresses some big issues common to most people who have chronic illness, as well as their caregivers. Joanne gives practical and insightful suggestions to help them renew their sense of hope and purpose in the midst of their many challenges."

CHAPLAIN BILL GOODRICH
Founder and President, God Cares Ministry.
www.godcaresministry.com

Epigraph

I come to the garden alone,
While the dew is still on the roses,
And the voice I hear, falling on my ear,
The Son of God discloses.
And He walks with me, and He talks with me,
And He tells me I am His own,
And the joy we share as we tarry there,
None other has ever known.

--Lyrics by C. Austin Miles, (c. 1912)--

Disclaimer

I have tried to recreate events, locales, and conversations from my memories of them. In order to maintain their anonymity or protect their identity, in some instances I have changed the names of individuals and places. In addition, I may have changed some identifying characteristics and details, such as conversations, physical properties, occupations, and places of residence. Names, characters, places, events, and incidents are either the products of the author's imagination or used in a fictitious manner. Any resemblance to actual persons, living or dead, or actual events is purely coincidental.

Although the author and publisher have made every effort to ensure that the information in this book was correct at press time, the author and publisher do not assume and hereby disclaim any liability to any party for any loss, damage, or disruption caused by errors or omissions, whether such errors or omissions result from negligence, accident, or any other cause.

The complexity of depression is beyond the scope of this book and is not intended to replace professional treatment from a medical provider or psychiatrist. The author urges anyone who is experiencing symptoms of depression to seek medical attention immediately.

A Note from the Author

My friend, there is hope for you. It is not a mistake that you are reading this book right now. My heart has been burdened to pray for people just like you who feel this way. I believe that as a creation of God, you have worth and purpose.

One morning, I was in prayer asking the Lord to show me how to love those in my path who are suffering. He reminded me that the depression many of my patients experienced was from a feeling of uselessness. He directed me to encourage them that despite a long-term, debilitating disease, there is hope for joy and fulfillment in any present situation. Then the Lord rose up in my spirit and gave me seven keys to a happy and fulfilled life despite a disabling illness.

The seven keys are simple and are many times overlooked in our daily lives. When you practice these seven keys, you may begin to renew your sense of purpose. The beauty of these elements is that they do not require physical endurance, significant mental capacity, or a great memory. They only require a willing heart and spirit.

Please note that although this book may help encourage you in your search for purpose, it is not intended to replace treatment by a mental health provider, primary medical provider or psychiatrist. If you are experiencing signs of depression, contact a licensed professional that can treat your depression appropriately.

Here is a list of the seven keys:

1. Listening
2. Observing
3. Describing
4. Encouraging
5. Laughing
6. Teaching
7. Praying

Join me as I share with you the meaning of each of the seven keys.

Blessings,
Joanne Bracewell, APRN-C

Acknowledgements

To my dear friend, Carolyn Sharp, I can't thank you enough for the countless hours you have spent researching scriptures, your encouragement and support, and providing helpful insights for developing this manuscript. Your prayers have given me the strength I needed to press on.

To my Editor and Publisher, Sherrie Clark, thank you for your immense patience over this project by skillfully guiding me in each step of the process necessary to prepare this book for publication.

To Artist Charlotte Dively, thank you for your persistence to capture the book's essence with a beautiful watercolor illustration. And thank you Sharon, for bringing the cover illustration into full bloom.

A special thank you to Arlene Sikorski and Chaplain Bill Goodrich at God Cares Ministry. Your expertise in recruitment, training, and support of volunteers who share the love of Jesus in nursing homes has been invaluable. Your encouragement and guidance with creating appropriate content is greatly appreciated.

To my colleague and sister in Christ, Sheri Powell, thank you for your encouragement when things became overwhelming, and I was up to my knees in the dirt.

To my buddy, Nancy Barbera, thank you for reminding me that we must always hold on to the hope of tomorrow.

Thank you, "little brother," Peter Wagura, for your helpful input with my title development. I am honored to "soldier on" alongside you for the call of Christ on our lives.

To occupational therapist, Sindy Lofton, who not by chance, found her seat next to mine in church one Sunday when this book was just a few notes. Your early vision and encouragement to look beyond my writing and into the next step gave flight to my ideas. Thank you.

Thank you to my mom, Joyce Lucas, and brother, Jim Lucas, for affirming the memories I have of Dad and his legacy of giving.

To my daughter, Janel DeJesus. I am so thankful for who you have become and all that you will accomplish. Thank you for your valuable input. Your hands have touched every part of this book. They are even on the front cover.

Finally, a heart full of gratitude to my late husband, Bill Bracewell – although our tomorrow never came, and your work here on earth is finished, I would give anything for one last heart-to-heart over a cup of joe. I so miss your delight in who I have become.

Introduction

Before my dad died in 1999, he bravely fought prostate cancer for almost fifteen years. He endured surgery and painful procedures. During those times and when in remission, he continued to reach out to people in need. He and my mom filled baskets with food and treats to give to people at Christmastime, volunteered in soup kitchens, and had responsibilities as a deacon in his church.

Dad pressed on, knowing God had a purpose for his life until it was time for him to go home to heaven. Dad recognized his gifts and value, despite the suffering he endured. As he took his final breath, I'm sure he heard God say, "Well done, my good and faithful servant."

I am a family nurse practitioner and have practiced nursing for over forty years. Over that time, I've noticed that many of my aging, frail, or chronically ill patients have lost hope for the future. They seem to have lost their purpose and feel useless. Somewhere along the way, with their children grown and their spouses gone, they have no one and nothing to rely on to help them feel useful.

Some of my patients are so despondent that each night when they go to bed, they hope they'll never wake up. However, our final day on Earth is not one we are able to predict. Our bodies age, and as time passes, we look back and consider what we have done and how we will be remembered.

Chronic illnesses commonly found during the aging process can keep us from going to work, babysitting our grandchildren, or enjoying the simplest of pleasures like going shopping, taking a walk, or climbing stairs. When chronic illness keeps us from doing the things we enjoy and that help us feel productive, we may feel useless.

In my nursing practice, I've seen how my patients don't feel useful if they don't know their purpose in their later years. These individuals become depressed, despondent, and without hope.

Caregivers are also at risk for depression. The role of caregiving takes its toll on the individual. Fatigue, isolation, frustration, and an overload of responsibility results from the demands of caregiving. The overwhelmed heart without hope withers into a state of depression and thoughts of worthlessness. Some feel this way temporarily. Others may feel sadness and depression for months or years.

Have you had thoughts that you're a failure and that you've let down your friends and family? Have you wished you could go to bed at night and never wake up?

I want you to know there is hope. However, it is beyond the scope of this book to address prolonged feelings of sadness, lack of energy and the ability to enjoy life. In this case, it's important that you discuss these feelings with your primary medical provider or seek help from an emergency room or licensed mental health provider.

Contents

Acknowledgements xi

Introduction xv

Chapter 1: Listening... 1

Chapter 2: Observing 9

Chapter 3: Describing 21

Chapter 4: Encouraging 33

Chapter 5: Laughter 39

Chapter 6: Teaching...47

Chapter 7: Praying 57

Chapter 8: There Is Hope 67

Chapter 9: What Next?...73

About the Author: Joanne Bracewell..........................77

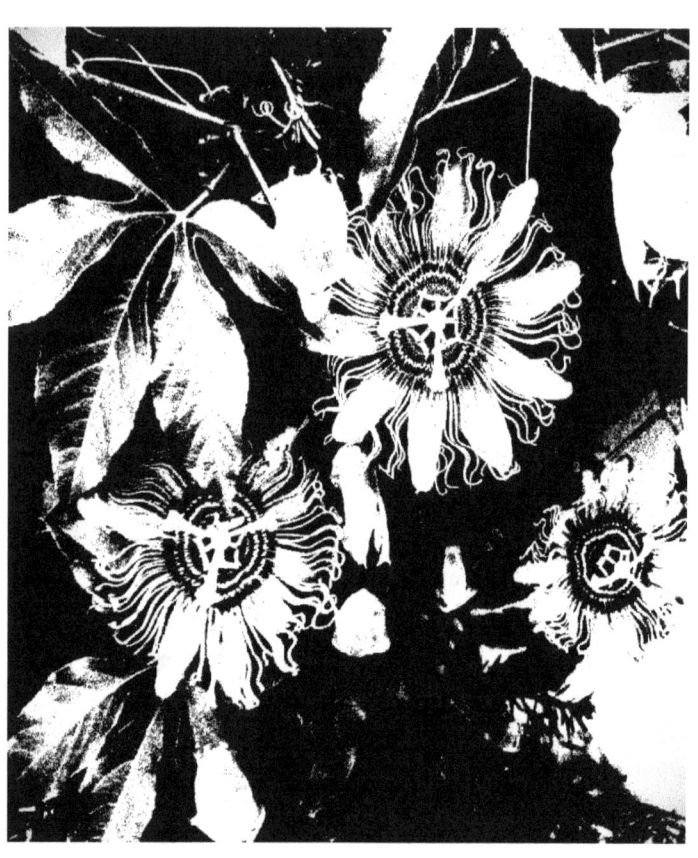

Chapter One

LISTENING

We all love to be heard by another person. When we share what's in our heart or our mind, and someone listens, it is as if someone has turned on a light. The window to our thoughts opens, allowing the light of connection with another person to lift our spirits.

No longer will we be alone with our thoughts of joy, sadness, or anger. Instead, we share moments with another person that may need our listening ear more than we know.

Of course, it's important to remember that listening to someone with no one to talk to takes a little patience. It's possible you are the first person in months who has taken the time to sit and listen. The flood of their words may seem overwhelming. It's not necessary to respond to everything they say. Just listen and nod.

Now, if you are the type of person who is wrapped up in their own suffering, listening and reflecting what someone shares with you can give you a break from the negative thoughts you are carrying. When you don't know what to say, just repeat back to them what they're saying to you. This response gives the "talker" a sounding board that they may not have otherwise.

Listening and paying attention has been a problem with mankind for ages. This is not a new problem. Think about this; when you read the Book of Psalms and words of the prophets in the Old Testament, the first thing that preceded any important saying was "listen" or "hear." It sounds to me like the prophets were trying to get the attention of a distracted people.

Take some time this week to use your listening ear and get together with a few of your neighbors. Look around you at the people nearby. Do you live alone, with family, or strangers? Perhaps you're currently living in a place where you don't know anyone. Do you live in a large senior apartment complex or government-assisted apartment? People are everywhere but you have no one you can call "friend."

I suggest you invite a few people to your apartment for a cup of tea or sit near someone in the dining area at your residence that you've wanted to get to know.

Once you are able to take the time to sit and listen to your neighbor or friend, it is wise to remember that when you are a listener you need to be trustworthy. Listening to another person is a privilege. Your friend needs to know you are someone they can trust.

They need to trust that you're not going to share their information with other people. Confidentiality must be part of sharing the gift of listening. Violate that trust, share with others those things that people share with you, and they are no longer going to trust you. Others will not want to talk with you again. You'll no longer be able to share your gift of being a good listener, and once again, you'll be alone.

I pray this doesn't happen to you. I pray you become aware of your ability to protect the thoughts that you have heard while listening. I pray you are sensitive to keep confidential information confidential.

*****

In today's world of high technology, there is little individual privacy. Nothing in technology can match the human touch, being able to share with another person your innermost desires, sadness, or joy, and know that person will hold close to their heart the things you have shared.

How many times have we heard about someone gossiping about a neighbor during dinner or posting a critical message on a bulletin board that destroys a relationship due to betrayal?

The good news is that God is our inspiration for listening. God Himself is attentive to our prayers and listens to every one of them. King David experienced a closeness to God and was able to share with Him everything in his heart. Reading through the Book of Psalms, you will see that King David shared when he was thankful, afraid, sad or at peace. He said, "But certainly God has heard; He has given heed to the voice of my prayer" (Psalms 66:19 [NASB]).

If you believe in Him, God is ready to listen to your prayers too.

PERSONAL REFLECTIONS
YOUR GARDEN: LISTEN TO THE SOUNDS

It is dusk, and a gardener is walking in his garden in the cool of the evening listening to the sounds of his garden. Bees buzzing about the Purple Coneflowers and Black-eyed Susan's signal pollination. There is a rustling in the lettuce that signals rabbits are foraging for food along the fence line. And, the comforting sound of a water sprinkler showering the garden is pleasant to the gardener's ear.

I wonder if Jesus heard similar sounds when he walked in the garden after His resurrection? Fortunately, He wasn't distracted enough that he didn't hear Mary cry out when she reached the empty tomb. He was there ready to show her that He was alive and that He was returning to heaven.

How can we have confidence that God hears our prayers?

The Bible tells us that King David prayed to God and said,

"I sought the Lord, and He answered me, and delivered me from all my fears" (Psalms 34:4).

"Call upon Me in the day of trouble; I shall rescue you, and you will honor Me" (Psalms 50:15).

1. When does the Lord hear us?

_____

_____

_____

2. When He hears us, what follows?

_____

_____

_____

Wherever we are, there are sounds all around us. But most importantly, the sounds and the hearts of the voices of people God puts in our path.

3. How carefully do I listen to those around me?

4. Can I hear when someone is in distress, frustrated, or can I share in the laughter and joy of friends?

5. What can I do if my sense of hearing is poor?

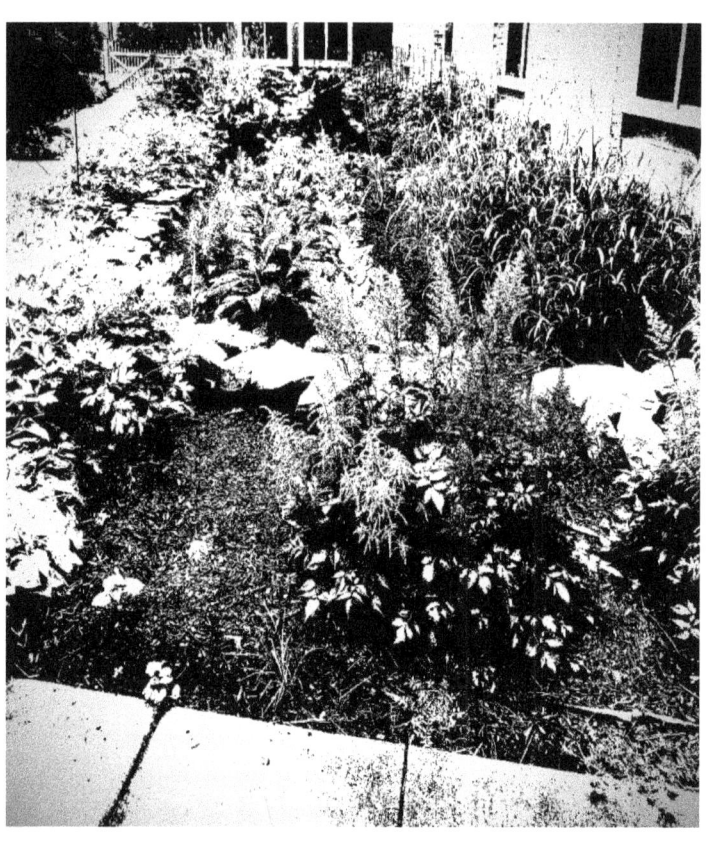

Chapter Two

OBSERVING

I have seen in my practice that despite poor vision or weakness in our hands or feet, anyone can make observations about what is happening around them. If you read this booklet or hear someone read the words, you can share an observation with someone.

Before you question the importance of observing, think for a moment about Jesus talking to the people in the Sermon on the Mount. Jesus used His observation of the natural world to make an illustration about having faith with these words:

> "Consider the lilies, how they grow: they neither toil nor spin; but I tell you, not even Solomon in all his glory clothed himself like one of these. But if God so clothes the grass in the field, which is *alive* today and tomorrow is thrown into the furnace, how much more *will He*

clothe you? You men of little faith!" (Luke 12:27, 28).

Jesus makes an observation with the intent to lead the people to a conclusion. If God provides the lily with outward beauty, we have every reason to trust that God will take care of us even when we don't deserve His blessing and favor.

The beauty of observation is that it does not require much physical ability to communicate an observation. We can use our hands, our feet, our eyes, or facial expressions to make an observation. Observing can be accomplished by using sign language, a communication board, or extending a hand to gesture to someone.

Nodding or tilting one's head forward can initiate an observation. Remember, though, an observation is something that requires thought and consideration.

Perhaps you can ask yourself: what would I like to communicate to my caregiver? What observation can I make about my condition that will help me focus on the positive? What conclusion do I want my doctor to make when, after making the observation, I feel she is in a hurry today?

Sharing thoughts about your surroundings could make an important impression on someone you meet today. It could be a description of feelings of the tension in the room, feelings of joy, or observing the beauty of nature. Making observations in your surroundings may draw attention to things that others may not have noticed. Making an observation can clearly communicate your needs and invites your caregiver to help meet that need.

Years ago, an unknown person wrote the words "stop and smell the roses" to remind us to slow down and appreciate life. It is a picture of how we can miss the beauty and fragrance of a rose garden when we are too busy to stop.

I work full-time, and I'm constantly on the go. However, I must discipline myself to stop and take time to focus on the here and now when I am with my patient. If I'm not careful to observe their actions, I could miss seeing an unmet need. I need to "stop and smell the roses."

For example, when I meet with a patient, I notice how they're walking, if they seem unsteady, or if one side of their body is weak. My response may be to help them obtain a walker. I also observe facial expressions. A patient who is looking down or frowning may have something to say. I can make an observation that I notice their sadness, giving my patient a moment to share how they feel.

Let's look at how we can put the art of observation to use in our everyday lives by looking at the following examples.

Food is a part of everyday life. Observations about the food that has been prepared for us can be helpful to our caregiver. Describe the taste, hopefully in a positive light. We recognize the value that each person has when we make a pleasant observation.

If the food is not to your satisfaction, if it upsets your stomach or is hard to swallow, describe the issue without being critical of the cook. Your goal is to use the element of observation in a positive way without attacking someone's identity.

Making a critical and negative observation can be destructive. Tearing down others by observing they don't fold your clothes properly or give you enough attention worsens your isolation. I have seen this to be true in my professional experience as a registered nurse working in nursing homes.

I knew I wanted to become a nurse after I worked my first job as a nurse's aide in a small nursing home. Several days a week after school, I'd work there until dark. Part of my duties included feeding patients. Paralysis from a stroke was the most common reason for their needing help to eat.

Some of my patients were appreciative of my help. It made me feel good to know I was helping my patients. But there was always a lady or gentleman who was critical and complained. I could never do enough to please them. As a nurse, caring for these patients was a thankless effort. I can't imagine how unhappy this unfortunate patient must have felt deep down. Perhaps if this patient had made an observation to me about their difficulties, my listening ear may have lifted their spirits. I pray you don't suffer in this way.

When your attitude is interfering with your ability to make an objective observation, you are in danger of becoming critical. Reach out to people as best you can and make observations that people can receive with joy. Even if you are unable to see, you can observe with your sense of hearing or touch.

Consider the lilies, the roses, and even the meatloaf on your plate. They can make a beautiful (and nourishing) difference in your life.

PERSONAL REFLECTIONS YOUR GARDEN: OBSERVE THE BEAUTY

A garden, full of life and growth, needs a caretaker to give careful attention to detail. The gardener observes the presence of weeds, the moisture in the soil, and blossoms that need to be plucked. Removing the weeds that steal nourishment, watering the soil and removing dead blossoms from the plants helps the garden grow and flourish.

Observing these things gives the gardener the information needed to sustain the garden's healthy growth.

The gardener in this illustration has been given charge over their own garden, but the gardener dares not to go next door into the neighbor's garden to remove a patch of weeds around their rose bushes.

Instead, the gardener may say to the neighbor. "Your roses are lovely. Have you noticed the weeds that are creeping in under the bush? I noticed it on my side of the fence." In this way, the gardener is making the observation with the intent of showing concern for the neighbor's roses.

1. How can I observe the detail in my life necessary to remain healthy despite my limitations?

_____

_____

_____

2. What can I conclude about my personal limitations by observing my surroundings?

_____

_____

_____

3. Would an assistive device help me move about or prevent my next fall?

_____

_____

_____

Jesus goes a step farther when He observes those who are suffering or in need of encouragement. He sees a need and shares His observation with his friends, the disciples, and is moved to compassion. Then He acts.

> "And Jesus called His disciples to Him, and said, "I feel compassion for the people, because they have remained with Me now three days and have nothing to eat; and I do not want to send them away hungry, for they might faint on the way" (Matthew 15:32).

6. What did Jesus observe in his circumstances?

_____

_____

_____

7. Who did Jesus share His observations with?

_____

_____

_____

Read verses 33-38. Although his friends, the disciples, were doubtful that anything could be done about the need, they pitched in and assisted Jesus. The outcome was extraordinary.

8. What resource did the disciples bring to Jesus to help meet the need?

_____

_____

_____

9. What did Jesus produce from their contribution?

_____

_____

_____

10. Can Jesus take what you have to offer and multiply your abilities?

_____

_____

_____

Ask Him to give you the faith you need to trust Him to use whatever ability you have for His purpose.

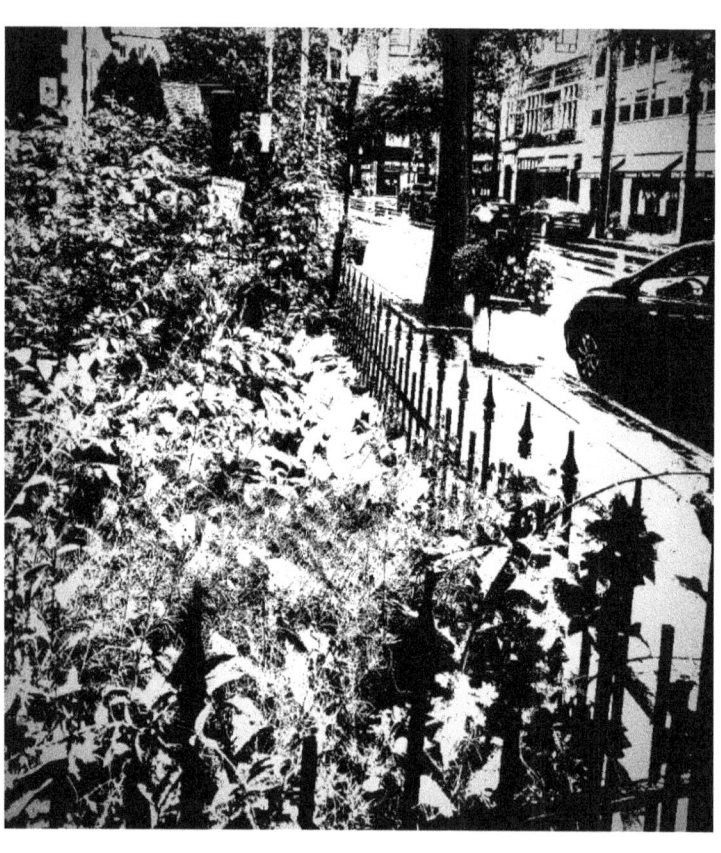

Chapter Three

DESCRIBING

We have discovered that making observations helps our caregiver to better understand our needs. We know that stopping to notice someone doing a good job or not feeling well shows we are looking beyond our problems and reaching out to others.

This next element takes observing to a deeper level. Describing is telling another person something in our own words, from our personal viewpoint, without passing judgment or giving an opinion.

King David wrote hundreds of descriptions in the Book of Psalms about the works of God, the beauty of God's creation, and all the things that God has done. In the New Testament, the Apostle Paul gave lessons to the new believers describing the events that would take place in the coming of the Messiah.

The Gospels of Matthew, Mark, Luke, and John described the things Christ did while he was on Earth. The stories of Jesus feeding five thousand people with a few loaves and fishes, or turning water into wine, point us to the power of miracles performed by Jesus.

The power of description is greater than just telling a story. It is one of our seven keys that can move hearts and minds because it tells others what they may need to solve a problem or improve our situation. It tells others the who, where, what and when of the situation.

I have had patients refuse to eat the bland texture of a pureed meal for good reason. Their description of the food's texture was enough information for me to act and improve the situation. If the patient hadn't described to me the unpleasant taste of the puree, I may have assumed they didn't have an appetite.

As a nurse practitioner and healthcare provider, I'm interested in knowing if my patient is in pain. I'll ask the patient to describe their pain and then give them some cues.

"Is your pain dull like a hammer or sharp like a knife?" This type of word picture helps my patient be able to narrow down what they feel. Can you make a word picture to describe how you feel?

DESCRIBE YOUR WISHES WITH A LIVING WILL

Another practical way to describe your viewpoint is to share your end of life wishes and goals of care to your family and caregiver. Family members and caregivers who share your later years will want to know your wishes and how to be prepared in the event you are unable to care for yourself. A chronic medical illness can worsen as time passes. If you need life support or you are near death, is your goal to remain at home or go to the hospital for extra care such as ventilators or tube feedings?

Describing what is most important to you when your condition worsens, gives your loved ones a clear picture of how to carry out your wishes. Knowing your desires in the event of an unforeseen emergency or accident will reduce any confusion with your family about your wishes for advanced life support. Avoiding future miscommunication with loved ones and being clear about your wishes is a gift of peace of mind that your loved ones will have confidence they are carrying out your wishes.

IT'S NOT ALWAYS EASY TO PUT WORDS TO OUR THOUGHTS

Describing tells others what they may need to know help us improve our situation. But sharing our thoughts with another person and being understood can be a challenge. Sometimes it can be difficult to get our point across. Have you ever heard yourself say to someone, "You're not listening to me?"

You are not alone. Consider Sarah's situation. Sarah was feeling lonely and wished her children would visit more frequently. One Sunday, her daughter, Jane, surprised her and comes for a visit. As soon as her daughter took off her coat and sat down, Sarah began to scold her.

"You never come to see me. Why don't you think I'm important to you anymore?"

"Mom," Jane replied, "I'm very busy but I made time to see you today." Her daughter looked away. Her sharp words hurt.

Sarah replied, "You don't listen to me. You've forgotten how much I did for you when you were a child."

At this point, Sarah needed to approach this differently. Instead of assuming her daughter wasn't listening to her, she needed to stop and ask herself, *Am I using "I" statements?*

Using statements that start with "I" show that you take responsibility for your actions and opinions.

When we use the word "you" instead of "I" in a statement, this tends to put others on the defensive and causes them to feel they're being attacked. In this situation, Sarah's daughter may feel that she is under attack. Once she is put on the defensive, she may shut down and look away.

What would happen if Sarah's description sounded like this?

"Jane, when I don't see you for weeks at a time, I feel alone and sad. I worry that you don't think about me anymore."

Sarah's observation clearly described her concerns. Using an "I" statement clearly describes what Sarah is feeling inside. Now, Jane can respond to Sarah's needs without feeling defensive.

It is easy to assume that others always understand our wishes. However, assuming your family or caregivers know your wishes leaves them in the dark to figure out what we are trying to say. Describing your wishes frees you to share your thoughts and be heard by others.

PERSONAL REFLECTIONS YOUR GARDEN: DESCRIBE HOW IT GROWS

Without a detailed description of all that's needed to keep our garden healthy, the gardener might randomly pluck healthy flowers or uproot the tiny shoots of a tulip bulb thinking these tender green shoots are weeds. Descriptions focus in on what is most important to us in our lives and protects new growth from being destroyed. There is great hope in sharing with our caregivers and family what is most important to us.

For example, a young mother with multiple sclerosis is suffering with severe muscle spasms. She longs to spend more time with her young child but is afraid to ask for help. If she doesn't describe how the spasms are preventing her from holding her child, will she find a way to solve her challenge?

1. What challenges do I have that need to be described to my caregivers?

_____

_____

_____

2. How have I prevented new things from taking place by not describing how I feel and what is most important to me?

_____

_____

_____

In John 16:16-19, Jesus was preparing his friends, the disciples, for a time that was coming soon when they would no longer be together. But the disciples didn't understand his prediction. Instead, they talked among themselves, asking each other what Jesus was talking about.

"So, they were saying, 'What is this that He says, "A little while"? We do not know what

He is talking about.' Jesus knew that they wished to question Him, and He said to them, 'Are you deliberating together about this…?'" (John 16:18-19a).

Jesus observed their confusion without passing judgement. Then, He continues and explains in more detail what he meant and encouraged them with a promise that someday they will have joy that no one will be able to take away.

3. When Jesus first tried to share with his friends about his future, how did the disciples respond?

_____

_____

_____

4. What observation did Jesus make to the disciples when He saw them talking?

_____

_____

_____

5. What or who do I need to observe in my surroundings so that I can communicate my wishes clearly?

_____

_____

_____

Ask God to give you the courage to describe the challenges in your situation to your friend or caregiver.

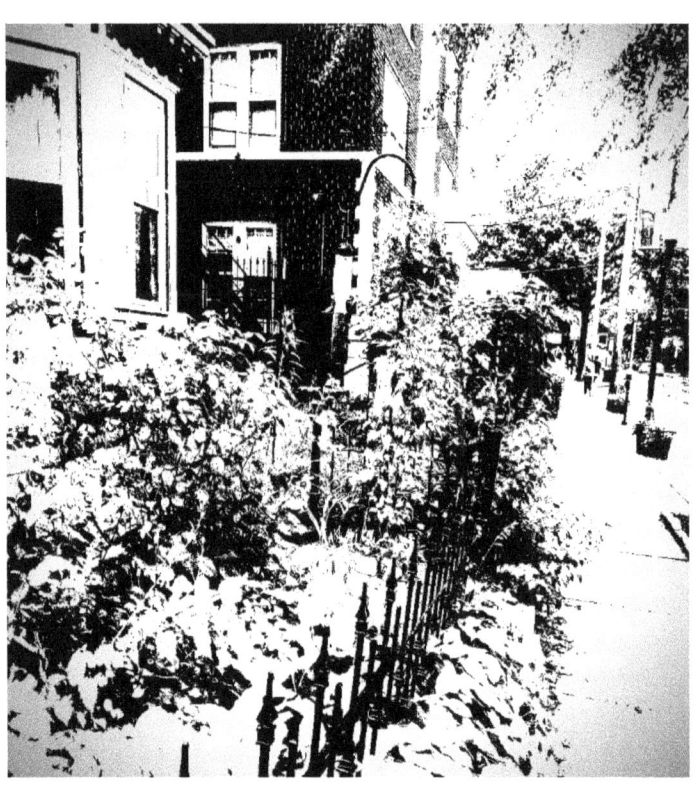

Chapter Four

ENCOURAGING

Encouraging other people compels us to think outside our own condition. Encouraging others to perform to the best of their ability, recognizing when people are doing something that takes effort, or perhaps recognizing that someone is doing something they don't really want to do, meets a need we all have for recognition.

Have you noticed an intellectually challenged person at the grocery store working hard to pack groceries with care, or the housekeeper who feels ill but still picks up the trash in the facility where you live? Maybe your nurse is having a bad day and doesn't really want to be at work?

Offer encouragement to these and others around you.

"You're doing a great job. I am so thankful that I have you in my life to help me."

These words say you're not only giving encouragement and showing appreciation, but you're also recognizing they have value and purpose in your life. Connecting with someone in this way is a way we can obey God's Word. Paul told the early church in the Book of First Thessalonians:

> "Therefore encourage one another and build up one another, just as you also are doing." (I Thessalonians 5:11).

Encouraging others to do all they can, to the best of their ability, will keep your heart and mind focused on making each day count for something. When some days are more difficult than others, we have humor to brighten our day.

PERSONAL REFLECTIONS
YOUR GARDEN: ENCOURAGE HEALTHY GROWTH

Although our garden can't respond to hearty applause from the gardener, people are known to enjoy regular conversations with their plants. It is not clear if the increased carbon dioxide the gardener exhales while talking to the plants promotes plant growth, but it's an interesting theory. Now, there are times when our gardener may need encouragement with caring for the garden if the day is especially hot or the work is heavy.

No doubt, it's difficult to work outside in the heat. If you've ever had to work outside in the heat or carry heavy bags of topsoil, you know how difficult gardening can be. So, when you see your neighbor outside, struggling with a 20-pound bag of fertilizer, you know their pain, so to speak.

Do you realize that the God of the universe, is also "…the God and Father of our Lord Jesus Christ, the Father of mercies and God of all comfort, who comforts us in all our affliction so that we will be able to comfort those who are in any affliction with the comfort with which we ourselves are comforted by God" (II Corinthians 1:3-4).

God knows about all our personal struggles. He comforts and encourages us so that we can extend that comfort to others. This assures us that there is purpose in everything, joy or affliction, as we go through life.

1. What two words does the writer of these verses use to describe Father God?

_____

_____

_____

2. What purpose has God shown me during my suffering?

_____

_____

_____

3. How can I use encouragement with others in my surroundings that will promote growth in their lives?

_____

_____

_____

Ask God to show you the people in your life that need encouragement today.

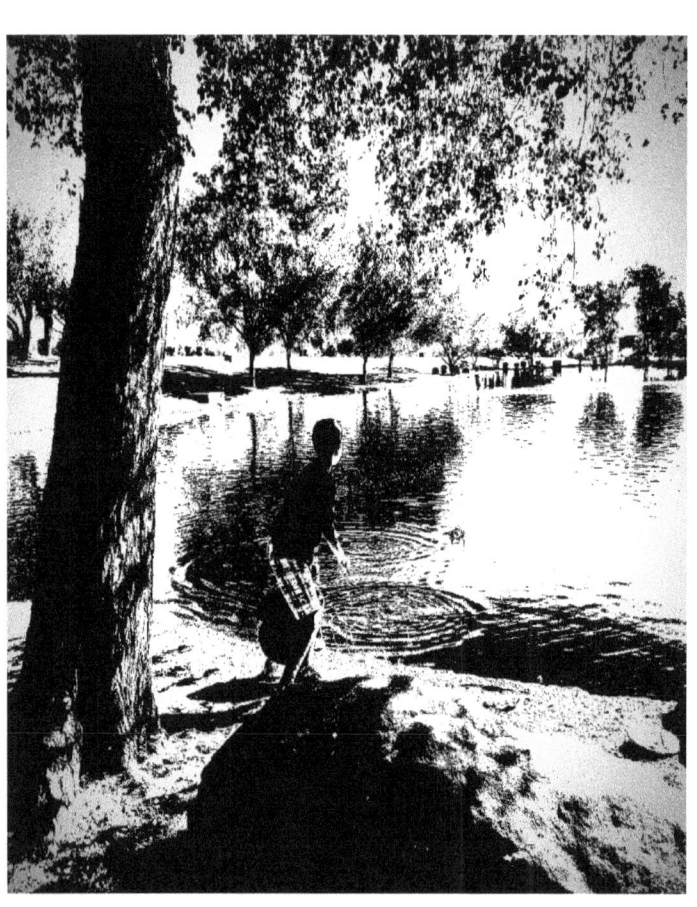

Chapter Five

LAUGHTER

Laughter in humor lifts the spirit and brings an escape from sadness and negative emotions that drain our energy. Laughter is a wonderful way to share the gift of joy with another person. If you have a sense of humor, this is a wonderful opportunity for you to reach out to others, share a humorous point of view and lift their spirits.

I remember my dad writing poetry and funny letters to his nurses and posting them over his hospital bed. Even though he suffered from the effects of his cancer treatments, he brought fun and laughter to his caregivers and physicians. What a testimony to God's promise that He goes before us and gives us peace and joy no matter our suffering.

Bring joy to those around you each day. When you have brought joy to someone, observing their response will be priceless. You may have a gift for being silly, for writing poetry, or wearing an outrageous, colorful outfit. Have you ever thought to wear something colorful to a doctor's appointment, put on a pair of funny glasses, or try on a new hat?

I fondly remember one of my aunts, who had a great sense of humor. Before she died a couple of years ago, she began to wear hats. Wherever she went, she wore a hat, and she wore it with confidence. She'd laugh or joke with people she met in the store or on a sidewalk.

I believe she used her hat to convey joy to people. She wanted to bring joy wherever she went. I knew when I met her at the airport, she'd be chatting with the busboy or airline staff, making them smile.

The more brightly colored the hat, the more she was noticed. Whether positive or negative, her hat was her signature of confidence and a joy-filled life.

The Word of God, the Bible, talks about joy and laughter:

> "A joyful heart is good medicine, but a broken spirit dries up the bones" (Proverbs 17:22).

Laughter is so good for our health. Did you ever imagine that laughter might prevent osteoporosis?

The Levites were teaching the Israelites what God's Word meant as they read the Law to them. The people were sad because they realized they had broken God's law. But then Ezra, Nehemiah, and all the Levites told the people,

> "…for *this* day is holy to our Lord. Do not be grieved, for the joy of the Lord is your strength" (Nehemiah 8:10b).

Passing on the joy we have to others is not only obeying God, but it is our source of strength as well. This is wonderful news. Friend, would you like the joy of the Lord to be your strength?

PERSONAL REFLECTIONS
YOUR GARDEN: A PLACE OF JOY AND LAUGHTER

Our gardener finds humor in the little things he sees in his garden. The ant that is carrying a leaf weighing many times over his own body weight. The cat chasing the mice out of the barn and the look on his dog's face when caught red handed digging up a newly planted flowerbed. Humor in life can bring humility.

Reading through Luke, chapter 18, we see that Jesus is speaking with people who had a pride issue. He used a puzzling illustration to explain a difficult lesson.

> "And Jesus looked at him (*rich man*) and said, "How hard it is for those who are wealthy to enter the kingdom of God! For it is easier for a camel to go through the eye of a needle than for a rich man to enter the kingdom of God" (Luke 18:24-25).

Imagine this word picture for a moment. A camel, hump and all, trying to go through the tiny eye of a sewing needle. Although His humor is tongue in cheek, the message is clear.

1. What message is Jesus trying to get across to the rich man?

_____

_____

_____

2. What humorous, funny things do I see around me that I can share with others?

_____

_____

_____

3. How can I use humor to get across an important point?

_____

_____

_____

4. What are the benefits of sharing laughter with others?

_____

_____

_____

Ask God to show you humor in the little things. Ask Him to give you the courage to use humor to convey joy to the people around me.

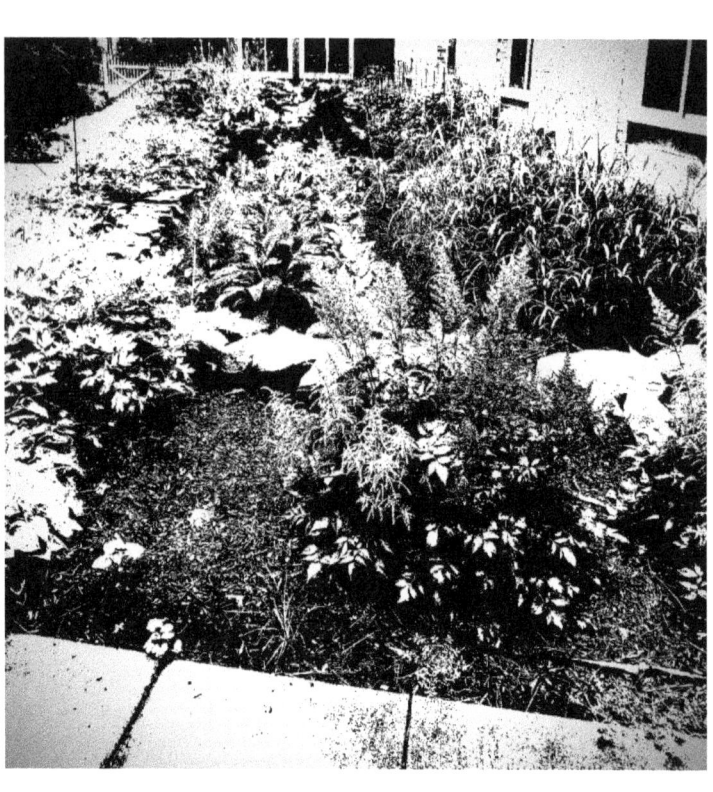

Chapter Six

TEACHING

Mentoring programs around the country have shown that people who share their skills and knowledge such as by volunteering in a hospital, children's home, or with a community group, gain personal satisfaction. Despite your personal challenges and physical limitations, everyone has a skill, knowledge, or personal history to share with others. Everyone is an expert about themselves. Have you thought about ways you can share your knowledge?

Sharing your life experiences in finances, success in marriage or parenting, contentment in being single, or even a skill useful for employment or homemaking are ways you can feel useful again. There are many men and women who have skills from past employment that can be shared with young people. These skills can translate into valuable employment opportunities.

Technology may be changing rapidly, but don't forget the importance of passing on the principle of a good work ethic. The foundations of wisdom and good judgment you can provide are valuable lessons for a young person to learn. You may be able to teach them how to be a skilled car mechanic, but if they don't show up for work on time, they won't be employed for long.

There are other examples of skills and knowledge we can pass onto others. Teach someone a hobby, such as woodworking or needlecraft. Teach children Bible stories, tell about your war experiences, or cultural and family traditions. These examples are just a few of the many opportunities to share what you know.

I've had years of experience teaching several levels of nursing students. I've taught first-year students how to make their first hospital bed – tight corners and all – and mentored experienced nurses who were studying to become nurse practitioners. I've learned so much from those moments. However, some of the most valuable experiences I've learned were from my patients.

I remember as a very young nursing student going to the home of a patient who'd had a colostomy. I had very little experience with caring for colostomy patients at the time. A colostomy is an artificial opening in the patient's abdomen covered by a special bandage. I knew that colostomy care is personal, and the patient is the expert. I asked him to share with me what method of care worked best for him. He was kind enough to show me all he knew about caring for his colostomy.

The experience was valuable for both of us. He had the opportunity to share what he knew with this young, inexperienced nurse. In turn, I gained a new understanding of the process that helped me to expand my knowledge of colostomy care.

Perhaps you struggle with communicating with your healthcare provider or caregiver. Consider that you're spending your time with them as a teacher, instructing them how you take your medication, what numbers you get on your blood glucose machine, or how you rate your pain.

As a nurse practitioner, it's important to get my patients' views on how well they are managing their health conditions. Your input about your diabetes or high blood pressure can be very helpful to a healthcare professional gauging your progress.

Do you have personal caregivers? I encourage you to share health information with him or her, using a gentle approach. Caregiving has its challenges. Oftentimes, it's a thankless job. Cultivate a working relationship with your caregiver that is mutually comfortable will give your caregiver strength to press on.

PERSONAL REFLECTIONS YOUR GARDEN: TEACH OTHERS TO GROW THEIR OWN GARDEN

Once the gardener becomes proficient at caring for his garden, he can enjoy the fruit of his labor. The pink flesh of a perfect ripe watermelon satisfies the Gardener's thirst. The green tasseled sweet corn appears on the gardener's dinner table that night. And, the gardener shares his bounty with his neighbors.

However, there is more work to be done. Now that he is skilled at gardening, the gardener shares his knowledge with others. He teaches them what he knows and prepares his neighbors to produce their own crop of fruit and vegetables.

Early on in Jesus' ministry, wherever He went, crowds gathered around him, desperate for His healing touch. He was moved with compassion and healed the sick, the paralyzed and the demon possessed. Once the crowd became too large, he climbed a mountain with his disciples and began to teach the people. He taught them how to live so that they would bear the fruit of being his followers and enjoy the benefits of God's promises.

Read the following passage taken from Jesus' well-known teachings in the mountain.

> "You are the light of the world. A city set on a hill cannot be hidden; nor does *anyone* light a lamp and put it under a basket, but on the lampstand, and it gives light to all who are in the house. Let your light shine before men in such a way that they may see your good works, and glorify your Father who is in heaven" (Matthew 5:14-16).

1. Jesus told the people who saw the miracles He performed that they were the light of the world. What was Jesus expecting the people to do, now that they knew this?

_____

_____

_____

2. What word picture did Jesus use to convince the people they needed to follow his instruction?

_____

_____

_____

3. What is the fruit or outcome of being obedient in this passage?

_____

_____

_____

_____

4. What things have I learned over the years that I can share with someone?

_____

_____

_____

5. How do I help to benefit another person's life by sharing my knowledge?

_____

_____

_____

_____

Ask God to soften your heart with a willingness to share your knowledge with others around you. Ask Him to show you what special knowledge you have that can enrich the lives of others.

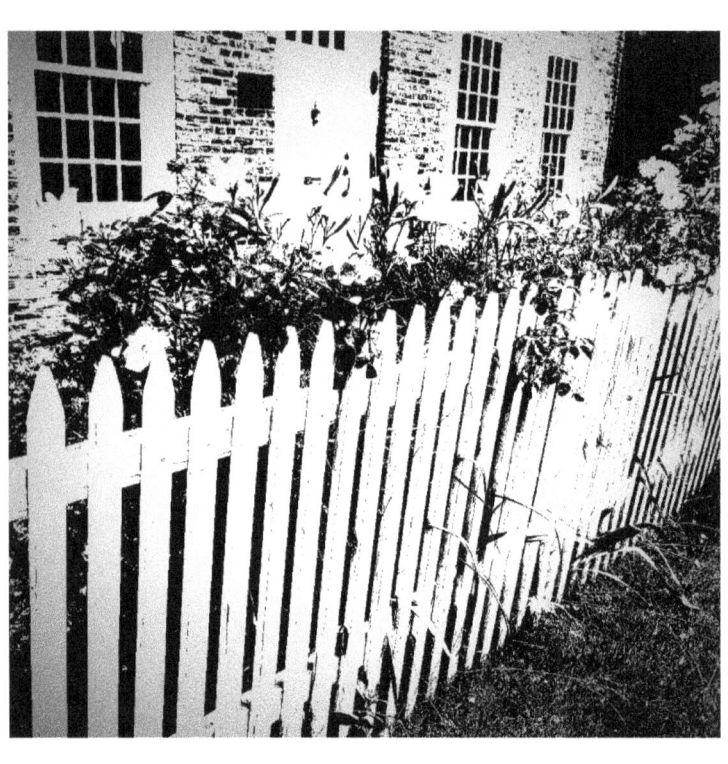

Chapter Seven

PRAYING

We encounter people every day who need to know that God is powerful, loving, and that He cares. You may find yourself praying for a neighbor, a family member, the check-out person at the grocery store, or perhaps a nurse who visits you in your home. The prayer of a righteous person, one who is in a right relationship with God through Jesus, is powerful.

Several years ago, I was the instructor for a group of young students in their first pediatric clinical experience at a large children's hospital in our city. Making my rounds, a student shared with me the clinical history of a young girl whose health was not improving. I felt moved to pray for the child. I stood quietly by her bedside and said a prayer of healing and health into her body. I felt the presence of the Holy Spirit at that moment, and I knew God had moved in her life.

Two days later, my student reported that the child had unexpectedly improved and they discharged her to her home.

Prayer does not always have a dramatic outcome in the natural, but lives are touched each time we pray. We can all pray for people if we have faith in Jesus and agree that He is our Lord. I've prayed with women in distress who experienced the peace of God through a simple prayer. You too can ask God to use you to pray with other people. The presence of the Holy Spirit in our prayer is powerful. He comforts, encourages, and brings our distress to Father God.

The Lord Jesus gives us many guidelines in the Bible on how to pray. The Lord's prayer is a familiar pattern for prayer.

Let's look at some of the things we learn about prayer from the Lord's prayer found in the Matthew 6.

- When we pray, the first part of our prayer is to give praise to God. "Pray, then, in this way: 'Our Father who is in heaven, hallowed be Your name" (Matthew 6:9).

- Next, we ask the Lord to provide our basic need for food, clothing and shelter. "'Give us this day our daily bread" (Matthew 6:11).

- Third, we ask God to forgive us for our sins. "And forgive us our debts (*sin*), as we also have forgiven our debtors (*others who have wronged us*) And do not lead us into temptation…" (Matthew 6:12, 13a).

- At the close of the Lord's prayer, Jesus gives praise to His father, God, for His all-powerful presence. God, the one true king. "…For Yours is the kingdom and the power and the glory forever. Amen" (Matthew 6:13b).

I have learned that the Lord does not expect us to praise Him for times of suffering. However, the writer of Hebrews 13:15, encourages us to "…continually offer up a sacrifice of praise to God, that is, the fruit of lips that give thanks to His name."

This means that we praise God for His qualities, *despite* our troubles. If you read the remainder of this chapter, God is pleased with this sacrifice and His ultimate desire is to work in you His perfect will. This is where I have found my true worth and purpose in life.

Consider these questions. How do you struggle with praising the Lord now that you are suffering from chronic disease? How can you offer a sacrifice of praise in your situation?

Over twenty years ago, the fathers of two of my children were diagnosed with cancer in the same year. Both men died that year, and by Christmas, I was thoroughly exhausted, grieving the loss of the fathers of my two young children.

I left graduate school, packed up the children, and headed north. I was a widow without the privilege of receiving comfort from extended family. I felt alone without hope that anyone would care about my situation.

At each funeral, few people knew that I was the mother of the children suffering this loss. God, in His mercy, showed me grace and His care through that time. His forgiveness for my divorces and healing of my shame were given to me through the promises He made to me in the scriptures.

> "Therefore, humble yourselves under the mighty hand of God…, casting all your anxiety on Him, because He cares for you" (I Peter 5:6a & 7).

"If we confess our sins, He is faithful and righteous to forgive us our sins and to cleanse us from all unrighteousness" (I John 1:9).

I realized that I wasn't alone, but God's mighty right hand cradled me with love through the pain. Consider these scriptures for you in your loneliness and pain. When you trust Jesus for forgiveness of your sin and accept Him as your Lord, you will know His grace for the difficult times.

*****

Sometime later, I found a wall plaque at a thrift store and hung it in a prominent place on my bedroom wall. The words on the plaque were the words of Jesus:

"The thief comes only to steal (*my family*) and kill (*my faith and joy*) and destroy (*my peace*); I came that they may have life, and have *it* abundantly" (John 10:10).

Jesus is explaining to a group of religious men who doubted Jesus was the Messiah. He explained to these men that He had come to overcome our battle with sin and Satan once and for all. This verse described so many of my life struggles. Even now, these words give me hope and purpose.

Considering all that I had been through, Jesus showed me that the suffering I experienced was a result of the effort of the enemy, Satan. I suffered from depression, rejection from friends and disappointed loved ones. The suffering brought me to a place of surrendering my agenda and the way I thought things should be for a life that followed Christ and His ways. I don't praise Him for the suffering. I praise Him for the fullness of life and joy He has brought to my life despite the suffering.

Friend, let us give thanks to God for His grace and love despite our chronic illness and pain. "pray without ceasing; in everything give thanks; for this is God's will for you in Christ Jesus" (I Thessalonians 5:17-18). Pray continually, talk with God about everyday life, and thank Him for His care for you. Pray and ask Him for even the simple things you need.

For example, someone who has had a stroke may pray this prayer:

"Lord, help me eat enough today to keep my weight the same. Lord help me to swallow without choking. Lord keep my hands steady so that I may reach out and touch the person you have put in my path. Lord, keep my feet steady and help me not to fall."

This humble and simple prayer activates the power of God, welcoming Him into your everyday life. As you experience His delight in meeting your needs, you will experience His love and care for you. How wonderful to know that the God of the universe cares to meet your smallest need.

PERSONAL REFLECTIONS
YOUR GARDEN: A PLACE TO PRAY

The gardener does his part to keep the garden healthy. He plants seeds, waters, and weeds his garden. But he also knows that the creator, God, is the source of sunlight, water and healthy soil needed to make his garden grow.

The healthy garden is a place of rest and reflection. Jesus went to a garden when he was in his darkest hour. He knew that He was to die on the cross the very next day. He prayed to his Father God to take this responsibility away from him, but ultimately, He was willing to be obedient to death despite his human desperation. Read Matthew 26:36-46.

1. How can I pray and tell God that I know He is at work in my life?

_____

_____

_____

2. How can I show God that I trust him with all that I am?

_____

_____

_____

_____

3. How can I show others that I know God has said my life still matters?

_____

_____

_____

_____

Ask God to give you strength in your difficult days. Ask Him to show you His light when things seem darkest.

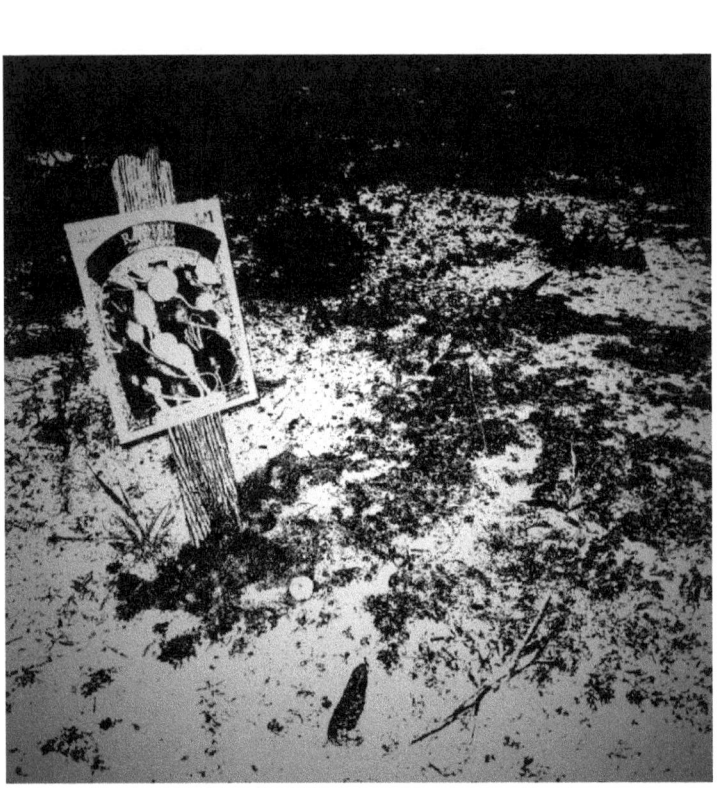

Chapter Eight

There Is Hope

Friend, I pray that you find this booklet to be of help and encouragement in your time of chronic illness or caregiving. Perhaps you are a caregiver, caring for a loved one. Your once active and strong father is now bedridden with Alzheimer's dementia. You feel helpless.

Some reading these words may have experienced the striking disability from a stroke. The right side of your face is distorted, and your gnarled right hand is a daily reminder of the stroke's crippling effects. Once you were an athlete and able to play tennis, or you worked in an office with charge over many employees. Now, you are isolated and alone or living with family where you don't want to live. It is more than you can handle.

Jesus wants you to have hope for today.

Our journey to rediscover purpose in life for today isn't complete without having faith in Jesus Christ and his resurrection from the dead. Sin (wrongdoing and mistakes) in our lives has separated us from friendship with God.

> "…for all have sinned and fall short of the glory of God" (Romans 3:23),

> "For the wages of sin is death, but the free gift of God is eternal life in Christ Jesus our Lord" (Romans 6:23).

But friend, don't be discouraged. There is hope.

> Jesus restored our purpose and worth in life by dying for us.

Thankfully, God has made a way. He sent his son Jesus Christ to die on the cross as a sacrifice for our sin. No longer will we have to carry around the burden of guilt and shame for our disobedience to God's laws. We are forgiven when we trust Christ and finally become free to live out our lives as God created us to be and then we can know our purpose and true worth.

If we rely only on ourselves to find purpose, we are limited by human abilities. Placing our trust and faith in Jesus Christ gives us confidence our worth and value is defined by the one who created us and gave His life for us.

"For God so loved the world, that He gave His only begotten Son, that whoever believes in Him shall not perish, but have eternal life" (John 3:16).

"Greater love has no one than this, that one lay down his life for his friends" (John 15:13).

The freedom of forgiveness through Christ's death makes us friends with God. To believers in Jesus Christ, the Son of God calls us His "friend." What more value could there be in life than to know that God is my friend?

"No longer do I call you slaves, for the slave does not know what his master is doing; but I have called you friends, for all things that I have heard from My Father I have made known to you" (John 15:15).

Now, my friend, would you consider taking a step of faith to finding your value and invite Jesus to be the Lord of your life?

Pray this prayer with me:

> Jesus, I have sin in my life and it separates me from you. I receive your forgiveness when you took my place on the cross to die for my sin. I want to trust you now totally with my life, my troubles and my plans. I accept your gift of forgiveness now and want you to be Lord over my life as I walk with you every day. Amen.

If you have prayed this prayer, ask someone near you to help you find other people who believes in Jesus and his gift of salvation. Find a bible and read it daily. Find others you can pray with to strengthen your faith in Jesus. Faith in Jesus as your Lord is the cornerstone for finding purpose, hope and value in life. Watch and see how the Lord restores your sense of purpose in this hour.

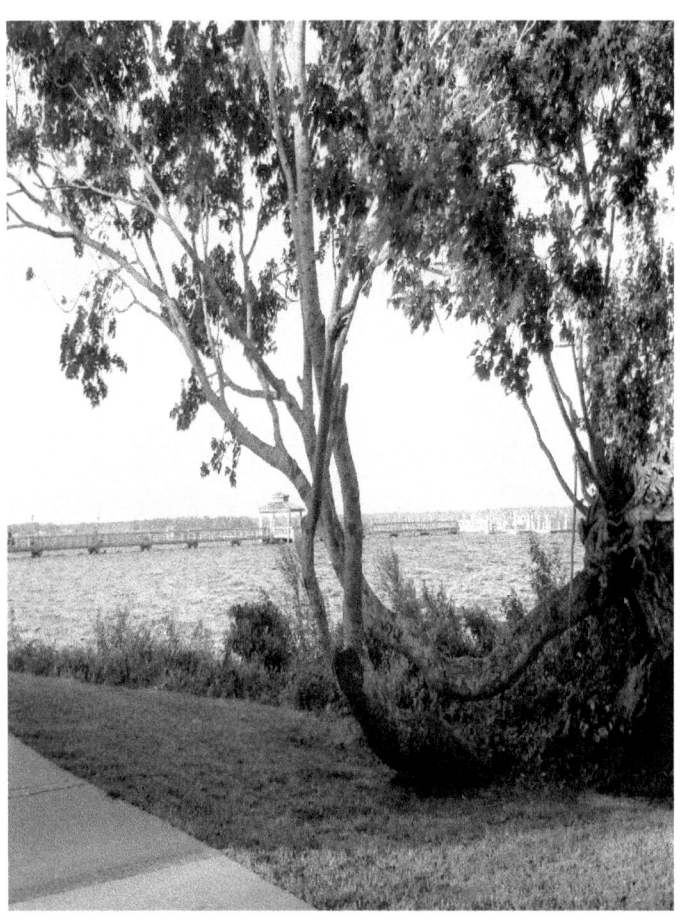

Chapter Nine

What Next?

Once we receive Jesus as Lord over our life and his forgiveness, another amazing thing happens. We are given a gift that makes our purpose in life clear. Before Jesus rose from the dead and returned to heaven, he promised to send the Holy Spirit to be a comforter and teacher to all believers. Now, you will never be alone. The gift of the Holy Spirit in our lives is the presence of God. Comforter and teacher, his quiet prompting of God's promises for our everyday life.

Jesus didn't promise a life of perfect happiness. He promised He would be with us always. God loves you so much, my friend. He cries when you cry and laughs when you laugh. He knows that your frail body, just an earthly shell, will not compare to the new body you receive one day when you leave this earth and go to heaven. You are created for His pleasure and delight, and His desire is to spend time with you every day.

Allow God to show you, through His words in the bible, your purpose in this new season of infirmity. Perhaps this illness is only temporary, and healing is coming in the future. Whatever the healing may be, becoming cancer-free, a normal blood sugar, or being able to sit up. May you receive your healing with arms raised high to God, giving Him the credit.

May God richly bless you in your journey through this infirmity. May He show you new things you would not have seen were it not for this infirmity. Difficult times are an opportunity to learn new life lessons. Continue to reach out to the Lord and seek Him with your whole heart every day. Ask the Holy Spirit to move in your life in a big way. May your joy, your value, and your usefulness in life be found ultimately by trusting in Christ as your Savior.

Allow the Holy Spirit in your life to create an atmosphere of love and acceptance to those around you. No matter where you are, show others in your actions that everyone has value. Understand that all of us can practice these seven keys as we age, so that we may walk in usefulness despite chronic illness or infirmity. Listen to others talk about their fears and their joys. Pray for your family and friends. Observe and describe your surroundings to others. Encourage those whom you meet. Share laughter and teach your family the things we have learned in life.

May God bless you on your new journey of faith, hope and purpose.

About the Author

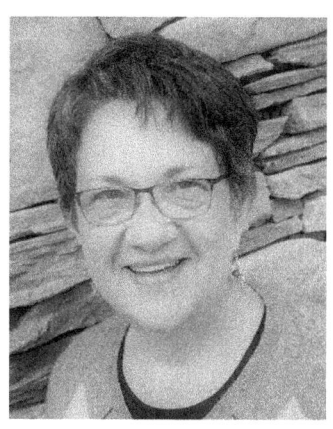

JOANNE BRACEWELL

Joanne Bracewell is an Advanced Practice Registered Nurse (APRN) certified as a Family Nurse Practitioner by the American Academy of Nurse Practitioners and certified as a Gerontological Specialist by the Gerontology Nurse Practitioner Certification Commission. She received her Master's degree in Nursing from Barry University in Miami Shores, Florida, where she was a Sigma Theta Tau inductee. Currently, in her free time, she is working toward a Graduate Certificate of

Completion in Biblical Foundations at Grand Canyon University.

She has over forty years of experience as both a Registered Nurse and Family Nurse Practitioner in the areas of mental health, family practice, nursing education, and community health. Her current practice focuses on geriatric clients in the community. She resides in Northeast Florida and serves in a county jail ministry and children's ministry where she attends Journey Church of Jacksonville. Whenever possible, she can be found enjoying time with her three adult children and nine grandchildren, who affectionately call her "Gramma Jo."

Joanne Bracewell can be reached via email at gracesongmin@gmail.com.

www.ingramcontent.com/pod-product-compliance
Lightning Source LLC
Chambersburg PA
CDIIW071722010410
42333CB00017B/2366